Green Smoothies
for Beginners

ESSENTIALS TO GET STARTED

JOHN CHATHAM

ISBN: Print 978-1-62315-098-3 | eBook 978-1-62315-099-0

CONTENTS

Contents

INTRODUCTION

Throughout history, the consumption of raw fruits, vegetables, herbs, and spices has been used as preventive medicine and to promote good health and healing, but for some reason, it never really caught on in the Western diet. And as people moved further away from unprocessed fruits and vegetables in their diets, health issues such as heart disease, cancer, diabetes, and strokes have radically increased.

The so-called "diseases of excess" are now at epidemic proportions. Fortunately, there's a simple answer for those interested in embracing a healthful lifestyle: put down the cheeseburger and pick up the smoothie! Don't cringe—the pages to come will show you how to make this delicious.

Curing your health problems and avoiding disease is really as uncomplicated as changing your diet. As people learn more about how their bodies function and what causes disease, it's becoming obvious that the key to living a long, healthy life is to eat right and exercise. Sounds simple, but that's truly all there is to it. In the course of this book, you will learn how to incorporate green fruits and vegetables into your diet in eye-opening ways that may surprise you—and you're going to love them!

What's the Big Deal about Green Smoothies?

The big deal is that they can literally save your life! Green fruits and vegetables contain chlorophyll, a special nutrient that you won't find in their brightly colored brothers and sisters. This will be covered in greater detail later, but for now, just know that your body needs chlorophyll to fight disease, keep your digestive tract and cardiovascular system clean and healthy, and fuel your brain and body. In essence, you can't live well without green veggies, as consumers of the fast-food Western diet are proving.

There are two reasons many people don't eat as much produce as they should: time and taste. It's much easier to grab a cheeseburger and fries or a sub than it is to sit down and eat a huge salad. No one would argue that chips are more convenient to carry around than a veggie plate, and a chocolate bar is certainly less messy to consume than an orange. However, in making these choices, you're trading health for convenience. Smoothies, on the other hand, provide a perfect solution to both of these excuses, being at once portable and delicious!

If you're eating a typical Western diet based on fast food, empty calories, and few nutrients, you're probably suffering from physical maladies such as energy crashes, acne, indigestion, constipation, and brain fog. You may write these symptoms off as the price of life on the go, but they're actually the first signs that your body isn't getting what it needs to function properly. Fortunately, there is a way that you can quickly and easily get all of the benefits of eating a huge salad without actually having to do so.

In the following pages, you will learn all about the health benefits of green smoothies and how to create tasty, green drinks to suit your taste buds. Not in the mood to be creative? No problem; you'll find simple detox plans here, along with tasty recipes for restoring health, energy, and beauty from the inside out. Getting healthy has never been so easy and delicious.

1

GREEN SMOOTHIES: WHAT'S ALL THE HYPE?

You've probably seen beautiful, skinny people carrying cups full of what looks like pond ooze and just can't imagine yourself actually drinking something that color, even though you realize it's probably excellent for your body's well-being. Well, you should know you're seriously missing out! As scientists have come to understand just how much diet contributes to health, the importance of eating a healthful diet has never been more obvious, and one of the easiest ways to incorporate more fruits and vegetables into your daily regimen is by tossing them into the blender.

There are about a million fad diets out there promising health and beauty, but most of them are garbage. Limiting your diet to only certain foods, eliminating an entire food group, or ingesting large amounts of one particular vitamin or supplement is almost certainly a recipe for failure, if for no other reason than the fact that your brain isn't wired to accept deprivation for long. The good news is that green smoothies aren't a passing fad, and they don't require you to eliminate anything from your diet unless you're on a cleanse—but that'll be covered later.

Green smoothies are simply an expedient, tasty, tried-and-true way to eat more fruits and vegetables—nothing more and nothing less. One of the many benefits you'll likely reap is that you'll find yourself eating less and craving fewer "bad" foods. This will occur because your body will finally be getting what it needs, and the fiber in the smoothies will make you feel full for several hours after you drink it. The result, of course, will be a slimmer, healthier you.

What Are Green Smoothies?

Green smoothies are exactly what the name implies: fibrous concoctions that are green in color! The more detailed answer is that they are made from whole, raw fruits and vegetables and contain at least enough green produce to keep the color of the smoothie green. Some smoothies are a nice lime color, while others may be brighter or darker green. You can drink them in a glass like a shake, or eat them in a bowl like a cold soup. The only rules are as follows:

- Use enough green fruits and vegetables to make the smoothie green.
- Blend it so that there are no large, chewable chunks (unless you like chunks, then feel free to leave them in!).
- Don't remove the fiber.
- Don't cook the produce.
- Don't add anything but fruits, vegetables, herbs, and spices to it. No sweeteners, milk, protein powder, or anything else.

That's it. That's all that there is to making a green smoothie. You can drink them for a healthful meal replacement, add them to a meal to boost the nutritional value, incorporate them as a filling snack, or use them to cleanse and detox, which will be discussed in Chapter 4. You've probably heard about juicing and may wonder what the difference is between a juice and a smoothie—to find out, read on.

Smoothies Versus Juices

There are two different ways to incorporate drinkable fruits and vegetables into your diet: smoothies and juices. The primary difference is that smoothies are made in a blender and contain all of the pulp and sometimes even the skins. Juices, on the other hand, are made by running your produce through a specialized juicing machine that separates the juice from the skin and pulp: all that's left is pure juice.

Why Smoothies Are Fabulous for You

Plants contain phytonutrients, live enzymes, vitamins, antioxidants, and minerals that people's bodies need to survive and thrive. There have been many civilizations throughout history that existed wholly on fruits and vegetables, and they were some of the healthiest people on the planet. There are no complex proteins in produce that your body has to break down for energy, though if you're drinking smoothies, your digestive tract will have to extract the nutrients from the fiber. The flip side of that argument, though, is that the fiber in smoothies keeps your digestive tract clean.

Why Smoothies Trump Juices

Though juicing requires a special juice extractor that can be quite expensive, all you need to make a smoothie is a good blender. Aside from cost, smoothies have several benefits that make them an excellent choice. For instance, if you're trying to lose weight, smoothies provide a ton of nutrients as well as fiber that will prevent you from feeling hungry. You therefore won't be tempted by those late-afternoon cravings that can throw your attempts to eat healthfully right out the window.

Another terrific thing about smoothies is that they're fast. All that you need to do is clean and core your produce and toss it into the blender. You don't even have to peel most of it; as a matter of fact, skins contain many nutrients that you won't get from the flesh.

Did You Know? *Many professionals contend that chewing is a necessary part of both digestion and achieving the feeling of fullness. If this is the case, then smoothies may be the better option than juices for healthful, gradual weight loss.*

Finally, some fruits and vegetables don't juice well, but you can easily toss them into your blender to take advantage of their incredible health benefits and luscious flavors. These include:

- Avocados
- Bananas
- Coconut
- Eggplant
- Leeks (You don't get much juice, and what you do get is extremely strong. Blending them, however, can lend a nice, mild, oniony flavor to your vegetable smoothies, as well as a huge nutritional boost.)
- Melons (Though you can juice them, you may get some pulp leaking through.)

The Benefits of Green Smoothies

So now you know why smoothies are so good for you, but what sets green produce apart from all of the other delicious, nutritious fruits and vegetables? The answer is simple: a little green pigment called chlorophyll. Often referred to as the blood or life of the plant, chlorophyll stimulates photosynthesis, the process that uses light to convert the plant's water and carbon dioxide into the glucose the plant uses for energy.

One of the reasons those in the know think chlorophyll is so good for you is that it's nearly identical in structure to hemoglobin, the part of your blood responsible for transporting oxygen. Some believe that chlorophyll can perform the same function in the body as hemoglobin. Though it's not yet scientifically proven, it's a viable theory, and there is some preliminary research to support it.

Other great benefits of chlorophyll include:

- Anti-aging benefits, including enhanced cell regeneration
- Antioxidant benefits
- Chelation of heavy metals from your blood
- Decreased inflammation related to certain illnesses
- Extracted toxins from your liver
- Improved cognitive function
- Improved healing
- Improved immune system
- Improved skin tone
- Increased blood alkalinity, creating a disease-resistant environment
- Protection from the harmful effects of environmental toxins and carcinogens
- Reduced chance of calcium oxalate kidney stones
- Stabilized blood sugar
- Stimulated bowel movements to help keep your colon clean
- Sustained levels of energy
- Weight loss promotion

These are just a few of the benefits of chlorophyll. As you can see, the reasons for going green are too numerous to ignore, but it's also best to get your chlorophyll from raw fruits and vegetables because heat—even a small amount—destroys chlorophyll. If you must cook your vegetables, steam them lightly; if you cook them to the point that they lose their bright green color, you've lost many of the health benefits.

THE BASICS OF GREEN SMOOTHIES

To make your first attempts at smoothie-making a success, there are a few things you need to know. Though making smoothies is a fairly simple process, making them taste good is another matter entirely. There's no doubt you're going to end up with a few nasty-tasting concoctions, so this chapter will also provide tips on how to turn a glass of "eww" into a glass of "yum."

Green Smoothie Guidelines

Before you get started, there are a few things you need to know to make your experience as "smooth" as possible! Remember—don't think of green smoothies as a passing fad or something you'll keep up only until you've lost a few pounds. You want to incorporate smoothies as part of a healthful diet for the rest of your life, so developing good methods and habits now will serve you well for a long and healthy existence on this planet.

Use Fresh, Ripe, Organic Produce

By using only the freshest, ripest ingredients, you'll ensure that you get the most flavor and nutritional value from your smoothies. Ripe fruits and vegetables have the most water content so will result in juicy, flavorful smoothies. You also want to use organic produce, because that's the only way to guarantee that you're not drinking a glass of pesticides instead of nutrients. Finally, it's essential that you use fresh produce, as chlorophyll begins to deteriorate as soon as a fruit or vegetable is picked.

Don't Add Anything

If you want to add water, spices, or herbs to your smoothie, that's fine, but avoid adding other components, such as milk, sweeteners, nuts, seeds, or oils. Remember that the goal is to obtain all the health benefits from the fruits and vegetables without complex proteins or other difficult-to-digest ingredients getting in the way. Introducing dairy, grains, simple sugars, or fat into your smoothie will interfere with your body's absorption of the nutrients.

Clean Your Blender

Cleaning your blender thoroughly after each use is vital both for health purposes and to ensure that the nutrients in your smoothies aren't compromised. It takes only a few minutes for oxidation to begin, and bacteria can start growing at room temperature in just a few hours. Take the time to clean your blender well each time you use it. Then you won't have to worry about any undesirables lurking in the cracks and crevices.

Clear Smoothies with Your Doctor before You Begin

There are certain people who shouldn't eat or drink too many greens or participate in restrictive diets. If any of the following apply to you, be sure to clear green smoothies and green smoothie cleansing with your doctor.

- Calcium kidney stones
- Diabetes
- Eating disorders
- History of allergic reactions to green vegetables or fruits
- History of problems with oxalates
- Hypothyroidism
- Pregnancy
- Taking regular medications

As a general rule, before you make any kind of radical changes to your diet, speak with your doctor.

Keep It Simple

It may be tempting, at least in the beginning, to add a dozen different ingredients to your smoothie, but it's best to keep it simple. Use just a few ingredients in order to keep your flavors clean, allowing your palate to adjust more easily to your new, healthful habit. Also, if you use only a few ingredients, it won't be such a struggle for your digestive system to digest it.

Mix Green Veggies Up

Alkaloids are chemical compounds that occur naturally in nearly all green vegetables but can be toxic if you eat the same green for a period of many weeks at a time. In order to avoid alkaloid build-up, eat a wide variety of green vegetables. You don't have to worry about your fruits, as significant amounts of alkaloids don't exist in any commonly eaten fruit.

Drink Your Smoothie Immediately

As soon as you make your smoothie, don't hesitate—drink it! The instant the skin of a vegetable or fruit is broken and air touches the flesh, the oxidation process begins, and the nutritional value begins to decline, so if you make enough smoothie to last all day, be sure to store it in an air-tight container in the refrigerator. A squeeze of lemon juice will help combat oxidation, and using a dark container that's the right size for the amount of smoothie you have is helpful, too.

Tips for Getting Started

Now that you understand the basic guidelines for smoothie-making, the next step is to examine some things you can do to make the actual experience pleasant as well as healthful. The most important part is to remember that this is your life and your experience. Find combinations that work for you, and don't be afraid to experiment. After all, life is an adventure, and your smoothies should be fun, too.

Make Your Smoothies a Rewarding Experience

Remember that this isn't a passing trend; it's a change in lifestyle. Keeping this in mind, make your smoothies delicious so that you look forward to them. If you like them, you're more likely to stick with it. Read on to learn some tips to help you make sure your smoothies taste great and keep you coming back for more.

Start with Transition Smoothies

Unless you absolutely adore the flavor of mashed spinach and broccoli, it's probably not a good idea to start with smoothies made from only green veggies. Remember, the only requirement for your smoothie is that it actually looks green. That means you can incorporate other fruits and vegetables such as pears, apples, kiwis, berries, or basically any other option to make the flavors more pleasant.

Use the 4, 3, 2, 1 Rule

You may find it helpful to use the 4, 3, 2, 1 rule of thumb when you're building your smoothie. Use four parts sweet juice, such as apple, pear, cucumber, or grape. Use three parts green veggies, such as spinach, kale, broccoli, and sprouts. Use two parts tangy or tart juice, such as lemon or lime juice. Finally, use one part zesty or spicy fruits, veggies, or herbs, such as cilantro, mint, ginger, or chili pepper.

Don't Panic if It's Awful!

Just about any combination can be pulled back from the edge if you know how to do it. Adding mild, sweet, refreshing, or zesty produce such as cucumber, apple, lemon, lime, lettuce, or celery can mellow out a bitter or grassy smoothie to make it palatable. You'll learn as you go, so if you make a few train wrecks in the beginning, don't be concerned. Chalk it up as a learning experience and keep blending!

Experiment

The best way to gain experience making smoothies is to break out the blender and get started. You probably have a basic understanding of many of the flavors that you're going to be using. In fact, if you think about it, you probably already know what many fruits and vegetables taste like together.

Use flavors that you're familiar with as a base, and build from there. Also, try the recipes in the following pages. Just because one may be designated as an effective acne drink doesn't mean you can't drink it if you have clear skin. There are multiple health benefits to be gained from all juices, so if one looks good to you, give it a shot. For that matter, step outside of your comfort zone and try something that seems a little bizarre to you—you may just find a new favorite!

3

CREATE YOUR OWN GREEN DRINKS

Your smoothie can be made from just about any fruit, vegetable, or herb you can imagine as long as the resulting smoothie is green. In that spirit, this chapter reviews several of the most common varieties of produce you'll probably use to get started. Since you'll already be familiar with their flavors and textures, your palate will have an easier time adapting to these in their new form. You'll also learn how much juice or pulp you can expect to get from an average serving.

Natural Sweeteners

These fruits and vegetables contain natural sweetness and will probably be the easiest for your body to get habituated to as you begin making smoothies. If you're having problems adapting to drinking your nutrients, try adding a few more of these to your blender until you adjust to the grassier or earthier flavors of some of your greener or less traditional ingredients.

Apples

- **Color:** Green
- **Yield:** 1 medium, cored apple = 2/3 cup
- **Flavor Profile:** Sweet with just a hint of tartness
- **Health Benefits:** Apples are rich in phytonutrients, called polyphenols, as well as antioxidants. They help regulate blood sugar, decrease your risk of asthma, and reduce your odds of developing several types of cancer, including lung, colon, and breast cancers. Be sure to core your apples, because the seeds contain traces of cyanide.

Apricots

- **Color:** Peach
- **Yield:** 1 apricot = 1/4 cup
- **Flavor Profile:** Moderately sweet, and sometimes a little tart, musky, and mildly "peachy"
- **Health Benefits:** Rich in beta-carotene and vitamins A and C, apricots help fight free radicals that cause eye conditions, such as cataracts and macular degeneration. They have soluble fiber that helps you maintain healthful levels of HDL, the "good" cholesterol, and insoluble fiber, which helps you to feel full.

Berries, Raspberry or Blackberry

- **Color:** Red or black
- **Yield:** 1 pound = 1 cup

- **Flavor Profile:** Rich, sweet, and sometimes a bit tart

- **Health Benefits:** Two more examples of health superstars, blackberries and raspberries are rich in phytonutrients called tannins, as well as copper, folate, magnesium, manganese, potassium, and vitamins C, E, and K. They're also a good source of omega-3 fatty acids, which help keep your brain and heart healthy.

  The antioxidants in these berries protect you from a host of diseases, including cancer and heart disease. They also fight free radicals and help prevent signs of aging, including wrinkles, dull skin, and muscle loss. The antimicrobial properties help keep you free of digestive issues, too, as well as fungal infections, such as yeast infections.

Cantaloupe

- **Color:** Yellow/orange

- **Yield:** 1/4 medium cantaloupe = 1–1 1/2 cups

- **Flavor Profile:** Sweet, musky, and refreshing

- **Health Benefits:** Chock-full of such nutrients and antioxidants as beta-carotene, folate, potassium, magnesium, and vitamins A, B1, B6, C, and K, cantaloupe not only adds a delicious sweetness to your juice, it also protects you from a host of illnesses, including macular degeneration, emphysema, fatigue, irregular blood sugar, low metabolism, stroke, heart disease, immune weakness, and several types of cancer.

Carrots

- **Color:** Bright orange

- **Yield:** 1 pound or 2 medium carrots = 1 cup

- **Flavor Profile:** Sweet and mild

- **Health Benefits:** Like cantaloupe, the health benefits of carrots are off the charts and would take an entire chapter to cover in full. They're a great source of vitamin A, beta-carotene, the entire B complex of vitamins, calcium, manganese, molybdenum, phosphorus, and potassium. The nutrients, antioxidants, and anti-inflammatory properties help keep your eyes healthy and promote good cardiovascular health. They also protect you from cancer, as well as prevent signs of aging, and do wonders for your hair, nails, and skin.

Grapes

- **Color:** Green

- **Yield:** 1 cup = 1/2 cup

- **Flavor Profile:** Sweet and tart

- **Health Benefits:** Chock full of antioxidants (about thirty in total!), manganese, potassium, and vitamins C, B1, B6, and K, grapes help protect you from breast, colon, and prostate cancers, cardiovascular disease, irregular blood sugar levels, and cognitive decline.

Honeydew Melons

- **Color:** Green

- **Yield:** 1/4 medium = 1–1 1/4 cups

- **Flavor Profile:** Sweet and light

- **Health Benefits:** Honeydew melons are a good source of vitamin A, potassium, vitamin C, copper, and B vitamins, including niacin and thiamin. They're a great way to help your body detoxify, and also protect you from cardiovascular disease, infection, skin damage caused by oxidation and collagen loss, several different types of cancer, and eye disorders, including macular degeneration.

Kiwifruits

- **Color:** Green

- **Yield:** 4 kiwis = 1/2 cup

- **Flavor Profile:** Sweet and tart

- **Health Benefits:** Kiwis actually have more vitamin C than oranges, as well as calcium and a host of vitamins and minerals. They have some amazing benefits, such as helping to lower your blood pressure, promoting circulatory health, protecting your DNA from oxidation, and reducing the risk of respiratory problems, especially in children.

Oranges

- **Color:** Orange

- **Yield:** 1 medium orange = 1 cup

- **Flavor Profile:** Sweet, zesty, and sometimes a bit tart

- **Health Benefits:** You probably already know that oranges are a great source of vitamin C, but did you know that they also have calcium, folate, potassium, vitamins A and B1, and several different phytonutrients, including anthocyanins, flavanones, polyphenols, and hydroxycinnamic acids? Oranges help lower blood pressure, fight off colds and the flu, and protect you from diseases such as lung and stomach cancers, arthritis, and atherosclerosis. In addition, they reduce your risk of stroke and heart disease.

Papayas

- **Color:** Orange

- **Yield:** 1 pound = 3/4–1 cup

- **Flavor Profile:** Mildly sweet, musky, and earthy

- **Health Benefits:** Though this brightly colored fruit is a bit of an acquired taste, the health benefits are well worth the adjustment. Papayas have a ton of vitamin C and are rich in vitamin A (including beta-carotene), folic acid, pantothenic acids, folate, potassium, magnesium, and vitamins E and B. They promote heart health, good vision, and a healthy immune system. Papayas also help prevent colon cancer, arthritis, and asthma.

Pears

- **Color:** Translucent green

- **Yield:** 1 medium pear, cored = 1/2 cup

- **Flavor Profile:** Mildly sweet, light, and a bit rustic

- **Health Benefits:** Pears have phytonutrients and are a great source of vitamin C and vitamin K. Pears are easily tolerated by people with food allergies, and they promote good eye health. Vitamin K is used by your body for effective blood clotting and to maintain bone health. Like apple seeds, pear seeds have trace amounts of cyanide that are released when you crack them, so don't put them in the blender.

Pineapples

- **Color:** Yellow

- **Yield:** 1/4 small fresh = 1–1 1/4 cups

- **Flavor Profile:** Sweet, fruity, and tropical

- **Health Benefits:** Pineapple contains the enzyme bromelain as well as manganese, copper, folate, and vitamins B6 and C, which help keep your immune system strong and promote digestive, eye, and heart health. Pineapples are also a great source of energy because of the sugars and B6. The enzyme bromelain is an anti-inflammatory that helps protect you from arthritis, cancers, and other diseases related to inflammation.

Pomegranates

- **Color:** Pink

- **Yield:** 1 pound = 1/2–3/4 cup

- **Flavor Profile:** Sweet, rich, and reminiscent of grape juice

- **Health Benefits:** Pomegranates provide a healthful dose of vitamins C and B5, as well as potassium, flavonoids, and other natural phenols and polyphenols that act as powerful antioxidants. Adding pomegranate juice to your green juice or smoothie can help protect you from several different types of cancer, heart disease, atherosclerosis, mental decline, kidney disease, and diabetes.

Strawberries

- **Color:** Red/pink

- **Yield:** 1 pound = 3/4–1 cup

- **Flavor Profile:** Sweet and nectar-like

- **Health Benefits:** Like other berries, strawberries are packed with antioxidants, as well as vitamin C, potassium, vitamin K, magnesium, iodine, and omega-3 fatty acids. They're great for heart health, including prevention of atherosclerosis, and they help maintain normal blood sugar levels, as well as protect you from colon, esophageal, and breast cancers. They can also keep you looking and feeling young by preventing cognitive decline, macular degeneration, arthritis, and digestive issues.

Sweet Potatoes

- **Color:** Orange

- **Yield:** 1 pound = 1 cup

- **Flavor Profile:** Sweet and earthy

- **Health Benefits:** Sweet potatoes are packed with vitamins A, C, and B complex, as well as potassium, copper, manganese, and tryptophan. These sweetly flavored, richly colored tubers are, in fact, even better for your eyes than carrots, while also helping to protect you from such illnesses as heart disease, diabetes, nerve system disorders, and hemophilia.

Did You Know? *Sweet potatoes have nearly 440 percent of your recommended daily amount of vitamin A in a single serving. Throw some cinnamon in and you have a disease-fighting powerhouse of a drink!*

Watermelon

- **Color:** Pink

- **Yield:** 1 pound = 1 1/2 cups

- **Flavor Profile:** Sweet, light, and refreshing

- **Health Benefits**: Watermelon is largely water, so it yields a considerable amount of juice. It's rich in potassium, magnesium, and lycopene, which makes it great for your eyes. It also contains vitamins A and C, and can help prevent breast, colon, endometrial, lung, prostate, and rectal cancers. It gives you a nice energy boost and helps keep you looking and feeling young because of the amino acid arginine. Finally, watermelon helps you avoid high blood pressure, type 2 diabetes, and erectile dysfunction.

Green, Grassy, and Fresh

Once you get the hang of juicing and your palate adjusts to the textural difference of drinking your produce in addition to eating it, you'll start appreciating the subtle differences that each fruit or vegetable can add. The grassy flavors of some greens may be too much for you at first—if so, just add in some cucumber or apple juice. If you want to go hard-core green, start with some of the lighter-flavored produce until your body adjusts to the delicious green freshness.

Alfalfa Sprouts

- **Color:** Green

- **Yield:** 1/2 pound = 1 cup

- **Flavor Profile:** Earthy but extremely mild

- **Health Benefits:** Alfalfa is considered the richest land source of minerals because the roots go down thirty feet deep in search of minerals. It boasts vitamins A, B1, B6, C, E, and K, as well as calcium, carotene, protein, iron, potassium, and zinc; it is also an anti-inflammatory and antioxidant. Alfalfa helps get rid of kidney problems in addition to assisting with arthritis, digestive problems, high cholesterol, urinary problems, and an entire array of other ailments. In other words—drink it!

Asparagus

- **Color:** Green

- **Yield:** 1 pound = 3/4–1 cup

- **Flavor Profile:** Green and rich

- **Health Benefits:** Asparagus is a great source of both vitamins and minerals and even contains protein. Just some of the nutrients found in this crisp delicacy include phosphorus, potassium, manganese, molybdenum, choline, selenium, calcium, and magnesium, as well as vitamins A, C, E, K, and B complex.

Asparagus contains several antioxidants, has anti-inflammatory properties, and is proven to lower your chances of developing colon cancer, Lou Gehrig's disease, cardiovascular disease, and type 2 diabetes. It also helps with digestive health, because it contains the carbohydrate inulin, which promotes absorption of nutrients in your large intestine.

Barley Grass

- **Color:** Green

- **Yield:** 1/2 pound = 3/4–1 cup

- **Flavor Profile:** Grassy

- **Health Benefits:** Barley grass contains four times the amount of calcium as a glass of milk, and as much protein as one ounce of steak. It also has about twenty times more iron than spinach does and is rich in vitamins A, C, E, K, and B complex. It has every amino acid that your body requires and is great for those trying to lose weight or get a good night's sleep.

  Since barley grass has so many antioxidants, it helps protect you from numerous conditions, including cancer, heart disease, cognitive decline, and digestive issues. Finally, it helps protect against signs of aging and alkalizes the body so that your immune system functions well and diseases such as cancer are unable thrive.

Broccoli

- **Color:** Green

- **Yield:** 1/2 pound = 1–1 1/2 cups

- **Flavor Profile:** Extremely rich and green

- **Health Benefits:** Broccoli has nearly every vitamin and major mineral as well as protein. It actually contains about as much calcium as a glass of milk, and is packed with phytonutrients that help support detox at every single stage, starting at the DNA level.

  Because it's so rich in antioxidants and is also an anti-inflammatory, broccoli helps protect you from several different types of cancer, such as bladder, breast, colon, and ovarian cancers. Finally, the beta-carotene in broccoli protects you from such eye diseases as macular degeneration and cataracts.

Celery

- **Color:** Light Green

- **Yield:** 2 large stalks = 1/2 cup

- **Flavor Profile:** Light, refreshing, and slightly peppery

- **Health Benefits:** It's not just a great partner to blue cheese—celery is a good source of vitamins A, B, C, and K, as well as potassium, manganese, calcium, magnesium, and tryptophan. It's been used for centuries as a natural diuretic, and also promotes arterial health, lowers your bad cholesterol, and helps keep your immune system strong by protecting you from free radicals.

Did You Know? *Because of its mild, familiar flavor, celery—along with cucumber—works as a great base for just about any juice.*

Chard

- **Color:** Dark Green

- **Yield:** 1 pound = 1 cup of juice

- **Flavor Profile:** Grassy and mildly sweet

- **Health Benefits:** The leaves of chard are packed with vitamins A, B complex, C, and K, as well as phytonutrients, calcium, iron, manganese, sodium, potassium, and copper. It's great for protecting you from anemia, osteoporosis, heart disease, cardiovascular disease, prostate and colon cancers, arthritis, cognitive decline, Alzheimer's disease, and high cholesterol. In addition, it gives your immune system a real boost.

Collard, Turnip, Dandelion, and Mustard Greens

- **Color:** Deep green

- **Yield:** 1/2 pound = 1–1 1/2 cups

- **Flavor Profile:** Grassy and earthy

- **Health Benefits:** These greens are packed with calcium, vitamins A and K, and omega-3 fatty acids, and contain lesser amounts of practically every vitamin and mineral. The large array of antioxidants serve to protect you from the signs of aging, cancer, heart disease, and other diseases caused by the inflammatory effects of free radicals. Greens also help keep your blood pressure normal, and the high amounts of calcium and vitamin K promote bone health, protecting you from osteoporosis and arthritis. Because of the oxalates in greens, be sure to switch them up!

Did You Know? *When you're preparing your carrots, radishes, celery, beets, and other root vegetables, don't you dare throw away those green tops! They're packed with many of the same nutrients—chlorophyll, too—as the vegetable to which they're attached! Toss 'em into the blender instead of the compost bin.*

Cucumbers

- **Color:** Light green
- **Yield:** 1 pound = 1–1 1/2 cups
- **Flavor Profile:** Light, mildly sweet, and refreshing
- **Health Benefits:** Rich in phytonutrients, antioxidants, and vitamin K, cucumbers are a great base for most any juice, whether you're using vegetables or fruits. They help protect you from cancer and other damage and diseases caused by free radicals, and they also contain lignans, which may help protect you from estrogen-related cancers, such as breast, prostate, ovarian, and uterine cancers. Plus, cucurbitacins, which are unique to cucumbers, block signaling pathways that some cancer cells need to grow.

Green Bell Peppers

- **Color:** Green for the chlorophyll, though all colors have amazing health benefits
- **Yield:** 1 pepper = 1/4 cup
- **Flavor Profile:** Sweet, green, and mildly peppery

- **Health Benefits:** Peppers boast significant quantities of phytonutrients and antioxidants, as well as vitamins and minerals, including vitamins A, C, E, K, and B complex, magnesium, potassium, and manganese. They also have anti-inflammatory properties that protect you from several types of cancer, including digestive cancers, and such diseases as arthritis, heart disease, and atherosclerosis. The beta-carotene in peppers helps keep your eyes healthy, too.

Kale

- **Color:** Dark green
- **Yield:** 1/2 pound = 1–1 1/4 cup
- **Flavor Profile:** Rich and grassy
- **Health Benefits:** As with other leafy greens, kale is rich in calcium, vitamins, minerals, and antioxidants. It's great for detox support at all levels and helps to prevent many forms of cancer as well as other diseases and ailments caused by free radicals. The anti-inflammatory properties protect you from heart disease and atherosclerosis, and the calcium and vitamin K work together to keep your bones strong.

Kohlrabi

- **Color:** Green
- **Yield:** 1 pound = 3/4–1 cup
- **Flavor Profile:** Extremely rich and leafy
- **Health Benefits:** Kohlrabi, like other leafy green vegetables, contains calcium, a wide array of vitamins and minerals, and large amounts

of chlorophyll. It's a common ingredient in weight-loss juices, and it's excellent for skin conditions, such as eczema.

Loose Leaf, Butter, and Romaine Lettuces

- **Color:** Light to dark green, depending upon variety
- **Yield:** 1/4 medium head or 1/2 pound = 1 cup
- **Flavor Profile:** Light and refreshing, and grassy with the greener lettuces
- **Health Benefits:** The greener a lettuce leaf is, the more chlorophyll and other phytonutrients it contains. Lettuces are packed with vitamin A and carotenes, which are fantastic for your eyes and skin. They also protect you from lung and mouth cancers.

   The vitamin K in the darker lettuces helps with bone growth and strength, and it fights off Alzheimer's, too. The folates and vitamin C are powerful antioxidants that fight free radicals. Lettuces are also a good source of minerals, such as magnesium, iron, calcium, and potassium, which help your body maintain a healthful metabolism.

Potatoes

- **Color:** Milky
- **Yield:** 1 medium = 1/2–2/3 cup
- **Flavor Profile:** Light and mildly earthy
- **Health Benefits:** White potatoes are known in the juicing world for their efficiency in helping clear up acne and other skin blemishes. They also contain vitamins C and B6, potassium, iron, and copper.

A special note about the vitamin C: You really only reap its benefit when you eat a potato raw or in fresh juice, because it's lost during the cooking process. Potatoes help support your immune system, promote heart health, work to keep your blood pressure low, and help maintain electrolyte balance.

Spinach

- **Color:** Dark green

- **Yield:** 1/2 pound = 1 cup

- **Flavor Profile:** Rich, grassy, and pungent

- **Health Benefits:** Spinach shares the same health benefits and nutrients as other leafy greens and is also extremely rich in iron, which helps keep your blood healthy. Popeye wasn't wrong when he said to eat your spinach—it helps keep your bones strong, your muscles functioning well, and prevents several types of cancers. In addition, it's rich in chlorophyll and antioxidants.

> **Did You Know?** *Spinach contains a whopping 247 percent of your daily recommended intake of vitamin A, which is a super-antioxidant that helps with everything from cancer prevention to fighting the signs of aging.*

Spirulina

- **Color:** Bright green

- **Yield:** 1/2 pound = 1 cup

- **Flavor Profile:** Extremely grassy and strong

- **Health Benefits:** This blue-green algae turns your drink a bright green and packs an amazing 60 percent vegetable protein. It's a great source of iron, zinc, magnesium, copper, calcium, and vitamins C and E. It also has quality beta-carotene and gamma linolenic acid, an essential fatty acid. Spirulina is excellent for helping protect you from cancers, heart disease, gastric disorders, inflammatory disorders, and other diseases caused by free radicals.

Wheatgrass

- **Color:** Green

- **Yield:** 1/2 pound = 3/4–1 cup

- **Flavor Profile:** Grassy and fresh

- **Health Benefits:** Wheatgrass is rich in chlorophyll and the nutrients found in the other types of grass. It helps to boost your energy, stabilize your blood sugar, and is great for detoxification and healing.

Spicy

Arugula

- **Color:** Dark Green

- **Yield:** 1/2 pound = 1 cup

- **Flavor Profile:** Peppery and fresh

- **Health Benefits:** Arugula has the same health benefits as other lettuce but adds a pleasant, naturally peppery flavor to your juice, while helping you detoxify and fight disease.

Cabbage

- **Color:** Green to milky
- **Yield:** 1/4 medium head = 1 cup
- **Flavor Profile:** Sweet and peppery
- **Health Benefits:** Cabbage is another superfood that offers a range of benefits, from cancer prevention to weight loss. It's used to treat ulcers and other digestive disorders because of its antioxidant and anti-inflammatory properties, and it also helps increase the good bacteria in your gut. Cabbage not only assists in prevention of many types of cancers but for some types is also used in their treatment.

Cayenne Pepper

- **Color:** Red
- **Yield:** If using fresh, you may want to limit your use to 1 small pepper per batch and adjust to taste. Powder is also acceptable.
- **Flavor Profile:** Extra spicy and rich
- **Health Benefits:** Cayenne pepper is a good source of antioxidants and, to a lesser extent, vitamin A. The capsaicin in peppers is a powerful tool used to treat ulcers, maintain cardiovascular health, and promote weight loss. It's also good for draining congested sinuses and is a natural pain reliever.

Fennel

- **Color:** Green or milky

- **Yield:** 1/4 medium bulb with greens = 1/4 cup

- **Flavor Profile:** Peppery and bright

- **Health Benefits:** Fennel is strong in antioxidants and adds a fresh, peppery flavor to your juices. It's rich in phytonutrients, vitamins B3 and C, potassium, manganese, phosphorus, magnesium, copper, iron, folate, and calcium. Research suggests that fennel can help shut down the signaling system that may stimulate cancer growth in your liver. It also helps you maintain good cardiovascular and colon health and keeps your immune system strong.

Garlic and Onions

- **Color:** Milky

- **Yield:** 1/4 medium onion = 1/4 cup. Use garlic by the clove to taste.

- **Flavor Profile:** Pungent and spicy

- **Health Benefits:** It would take another entire book to fully review all of the health benefits of garlic and onions, but perhaps most important is that they are fantastic sources of antioxidants as well as vitamins B6 and C, folate, potassium, manganese, and tryptophan.

Garlic and onions keep your immune system strong to help you fight off colds, the flu, and disease; they promote digestive health, help your body metabolize iron, which is great for your blood, and kill bacteria in your mouth that cause gum disease. And the big benefit? The sulfides and antioxidants are extremely anti-carcinogenic and protect you from a wide range of cancers.

Ginger

- **Color:** Milky

- **Yield:** 1 finger-size piece = 2 tablespoons

- **Flavor Profile:** Zesty and extremely spicy

- **Health Benefits:** The gingerol in ginger is not only a powerful antioxidant but actually stimulates apoptosis, or cell death, in ovarian cancer. It's also been used for centuries to treat stomach upset and disorders such as motion sickness. Ginger strengthens your immune system and is also great for reducing the swelling and pain associated with arthritis.

Horseradish

- **Color:** Milky

- **Yield:** 1 finger-size piece = 2 tablespoons

- **Flavor Profile:** Extremely spicy

- **Health Benefits:** Horseradish can add a deliciously spicy zing to your green smoothies, and contains nutrients, antioxidants, and anti-inflammatory properties that lessen arthritis pain and swelling, fight off colds and the flu, and battle cancer, just to name a few benefits. It's also excellent for respiratory and sinus issues, and promotes good urinary health. And as an added bonus, it's great for your skin and for detoxification.

Jalapeño Peppers

- **Color:** Green

- **Yield:** 1 pepper = 1 tablespoon

- **Flavor Profile:** Extremely spicy

- **Health Benefits:** Just as with cayenne peppers, jalapeños are a great source of capsaicin, and since they're green, you're getting the benefits of chlorophyll as well. They're great for digestion, and if you don't use the seeds, you can greatly reduce the heat.

Radishes

- **Color:** Milky and the greens are, of course, green

- **Yield:** 4 medium = 1/4 cup

- **Flavor Profile:** Peppery and spicy; the greens are earthy and grassy with a hint of spice

- **Health Benefits:** The biggest thing radishes have going for them is their vitamin C content. They also contain trace minerals, though not in significant amounts. Vitamin C is a great detoxifier and can help protect you from several different types of cancer, including oral, kidney, and digestive cancers. And as everyone knows, vitamin C is great for fighting off colds and the flu, as well as diabetes, cardiovascular disease, urinary tract infections, and kidney disease.

Zesty, Tart

Grapefruits, Lemons, and Limes

- **Color:** Pink, yellow, or green

- **Yield:** 1 grapefruit = 1/2 cup; 1 lemon or lime = 1/4 cup

- **Flavor Profile:** Sweet and tart

- **Health Benefits:** Tart citrus fruits are delicious and chock-full of vitamins A, B, and C. They're terrific for your immune system, and the antioxidants destroy free radicals that cause cancers such as breast, colon, lung, stomach, and skin cancers. They also contain the phytonutrient limonin, which keeps cancer cells from growing. Citrus juice can also help prevent certain kidney stones by lowering your pH, and it assists in lowering your bad cholesterol.

Lemongrass

- **Color:** Green

- **Yield:** 1 pound = 2/3–1 cup

- **Flavor Profile:** Grassy with lemony tones

- **Health Benefits:** Great for detoxing, because in addition to the other benefits of chlorophyll, it also boosts your immune system, eliminates toxins, boosts your energy levels by increasing the level of oxygen in your blood, and promotes healing throughout your body.

Tomatoes

- **Color:** Red

- **Yield:** 1 pound = 1–1 1/2 cups

- **Flavor Profile:** Rich and, well, "tomato-ey"

- **Health Benefits:** Tomatoes are fantastic for your health and also make a great base for creating a green juice with a familiar flavor profile. They're rich in vitamin A (including beta-carotene and zeaxanthin), B complex, C, E, and K, as well as the minerals copper, iron, magnesium, tryptophan, phosphorus, and potassium. And, yes, tomatoes have protein, too. They're excellent for keeping your eyes, heart, and bones healthy, plus the antioxidant alpha-tomatine interferes with the growth of prostate and lung cancer cells, and possibly breast and pancreatic cancer cells, too.

Watercress

- **Color:** Green leaves, milky bulb

- **Yield:** 1/2 pound = 1 cup

- **Flavor Profile:** Peppery

- **Health Benefits:** This zesty plant is both tasty and good for you. It's a natural diuretic and its antioxidants protect you from cancer. It has also been used for centuries as a digestive aid, and it helps with respiratory issues by clearing your airway.

Did You Know? *If you're taking certain medications such as chlorzoxazone, you should speak with your doctor prior to consuming watercress, because there may be an interaction.*

Herbs

Basil

- **Color:** Dark green

- **Yield:** 1/2 pound = 1 cup

- **Flavor Profile:** Bright and refreshingly spicy

- **Health Benefits:** Basil has the same nutrients as other leafy greens and adds an appetizing, familiar "spaghetti sauce" zing to your juice. It's currently being studied for its antibacterial properties, because it's suspected that basil can fight disease-causing bacteria that have become immune to mainstream antibiotics. Because it has such a strong flavor, be careful adding more than just a few leaves!

Cilantro

- **Color:** Dark Green

- **Yield:** 1/2 pound = 1 cup

- **Flavor Profile:** Spicy and grassy

- **Health Benefits:** Cilantro carries the same health benefits as other leafy greens and also helps control your blood sugar, while decreasing bad (LDL) cholesterol.

Did You Know? *Cilantro, also known as coriander, adds a flavor reminiscent of salsa to your juice, because it's the primary herb in that recipe. Like basil, cilantro is also being studied for its beneficial antibacterial properties.*

Dill

- **Color:** Green

- **Yield:** 1/2 pound = 1 cup

- **Flavor Profile:** Sweet and spicy

- **Health Benefits:** Packed with antioxidants, calcium, and antibacterial and anti-inflammatory properties, dill is great for preventing osteoporosis, infections, heart disease, cancer, and other illnesses related to damage by free radicals. It's often used with chamomile to promote relaxation and sleep.

Did You Know? *Dill has been used as a cure for hiccups and headaches for centuries. Just place it in boiling water, let it steep, drain, and drink the resulting tea.*

Mint

- **Color:** Bright green

- **Yield:** 1/2 pound = 1 cup

- **Flavor Profile:** Sweet, bright, and refreshing—a few leaves will go a long way.

- **Health Benefits:** For centuries, this delicious leaf—used to make candy for centuries as well as a digestive aid to calm upset stomachs—packs a huge health punch. It contains antioxidants that fight cancer and is loaded with antimicrobial oils that kill such bad bacteria as salmonella, E. coli, and staph. Mint is also great for respiratory problems related to inflammation, such as allergies and asthma.

Parsley

- **Color:** Bright green
- **Yield:** 1 pound = 2/3–1 cup
- **Flavor Profile:** Grassy and vibrant
- **Health Benefits:** Parsley contains all of the benefits of other leafy greens, as well as volatile oils that have been shown to slow down tumor formation, particularly in the lungs. It's also rich in flavonoids, or antioxidants that fight free radicals and reduce your chances of getting cancer, including colon cancer. In addition, parsley reduces your odds of contracting such diseases as diabetes, asthma, heart disease, and atherosclerosis.

Spices

Cinnamon

- **Color:** Red or brown
- **Yield:** Use store-bought powder or freshly grind a stick at home
- **Flavor Profile:** Spicy and woodsy
- **Health Benefits:** This aromatic herb that reminds many people of the holidays is packed with antioxidants and anti-inflammatory properties that help you maintain heart, colon, and immune health. It also helps regulate your metabolism and blood sugar levels and is a natural antibacterial and antifungal. Throw this into your juice for a healthful burst of flavor!

Clove

- **Color:** Brown

- **Yield:** Use store-bought powder or dried whole cloves

- **Flavor Profile:** Spicy, sweet, and woodsy

- **Health Benefits:** Cloves contain more antioxidants than any other ingredient, and therefore constitute an amazing addition to your juices. They blend well with both ginger and cinnamon, so feel free to throw them into drinks in which you're using those spices, too. Cloves also have antiseptic, anti-inflammatory, and germicidal properties, so they're great for heading off the flu, infections, arthritis, and digestive issues. Because of their high antioxidant content, cloves help your body fight everything from colds to cancer, so use them liberally!

Turmeric

- **Color:** Bright Orange

- **Yield:** The actual root is pretty hard to find fresh, so just use it in powder form

- **Flavor Profile:** Spicy and slightly ginger-like

- **Health Benefits:** The benefits of this orange cousin of ginger are about as long as your arm, so here are just the most important ones. Turmeric doesn't just fight free radicals to prevent cancer, it actually blocks the enzyme that promotes its growth. It may also be useful in the actual treatment of certain cancers, including colon, prostate, and skin cancers. It's an amazing anti-inflammatory as well and is therefore beneficial to those with arthritis.

This is only a list of some of the most popular fruits, vegetables, herbs, and spices. Just because it's not on the list doesn't mean that you can't use it or that it won't be good. Basically, if it's green, leafy, and grows, throw it into your blender one ingredient at a time and see how it goes—you can always add in some apple or cucumber juice to level it back out!

Tips for Creating Your Own Smoothies

As you get comfortable making smoothies and learn which flavors work well together, you're going to want to strike out on your own and start creating unique, delicious concoctions. That's great, and here are a few tips to keep you on track as you develop all new flavor profiles based upon your goals and preferences.

Start with a Neutral Base

Vegetables such as tomatoes, lettuce, and cucumbers offer a familiar base that blends well with most any other vegetable or even fruit. If you start with these in the beginning, your attempt at creating a great-tasting smoothie is off to a good start.

Try Adding New Flavors to Familiar Ones

You have a general idea of what most produce tastes like, so get creative and start adding new ingredients to your base mixes. If you love the flavors of tomato, basil, pepper, and cucumber, try tossing in some celery to see what you think. Use a small amount at first and taste as you add. Before you know it, you'll have a whole new arsenal of flavors!

Taste As You Go

Trying new flavors together is the only way that you're going to discover new recipes, but add a little bit at a time when you're creating a new masterpiece, and taste as you go. You may be surprised how much just a teaspoon of horseradish, half a jalapeño, or a few leaves of basil can change your flavor profiles. It's easy to add more "kick," but not so simple to correct once it's so spicy you could strip paint with it!

Get a Little Crazy with It!

Flavors you think sound completely unappealing together may just turn out to be some of your favorites! Try a little cayenne in your fruit smoothies or a leaf or two of mint in your veggie juice. You never know until you try.

This chapter covered the benefits of incorporating smoothies into your daily diet, but what if you want to cleanse and detoxify your body by undergoing a green smoothie detox? A smoothie detox isn't quite as drastic as a juice cleanse, but there are still some side effects of which you should be aware. However, a good cleanse can really get your body back on track. The next chapter presents how to properly undergo a detox, what the health benefits are, and what types of side effects you might expect.

4

WHAT IS A CLEANSE?

You hear about them all the time: cleanses, detox plans, juice fasts. But really, what are they? Though many people use these terms interchangeably, they're not the same at all. Juicing involves removing the juice from your produce and drinking it, while discarding the pulp. A smoothie, on the other hand, contains both the juice and the pulp.

Before covering the details of your impending smoothie cleanse, the differences between a detox and a cleanse need to be clarified. Most people think that they're the same thing, when they are in fact two very different practices.

- **Detox:** If you want to eliminate all of the toxins from your system, you do a detox. The goal is to eliminate heavy metals, cigarette toxins, and environmental toxins that you come into contact with via touch or breathing, chemicals that you may absorb from cleaning agents or chemicals, and just about any other foreign, toxic substance that may be floating around in your bloodstream just waiting to make you sick.

Since your main goal here is healing, you may want to use juice to detox because it makes digestion simple; your digestive tract

43

doesn't have to extract the nutrients from fiber, and the energy saved can be used for healing.

- **Cleanse:** If you want to clean out your digestive tract from top to bottom of all toxins, parasites, lingering fecal matter, or fungi such as candida, then you'll want to do a cleanse. Smoothies are great for cleansing because the fiber in the produce sweeps all of this junk right out of your system, while the phytonutrients and antioxidants in the plants work to heal you and fight disease and free radicals that cause sickness and aging.

Another difference is that in order to be considered a true detox, most people will say you need to eliminate fiber from your diet, so your body can focus on healing instead of digestion.

So what are the advantages of doing a smoothie cleanse versus a juice fast or detox? There are several, but which one is better for you depends entirely upon your personal health and your goals. The primary difference is that since you are still eating fiber, your body isn't getting the mad rush of nutrients that can initially cause nausea, vomiting, and headaches in people new to juicing.

How to Prepare for Your Cleanse

A smoothie cleanse isn't quite as traumatic to your system as a juice detox because you are still consuming fiber; even so, you'll want to prepare your body for the change in order to lessen or avoid the side effects. Here are a few tips that will help make your transition to a smoothie-only diet a little bit easier.

- Stop smoking two weeks before your cleanse.

- Eliminate dairy, simple sugars, caffeine, and processed foods three days prior to cleansing.

- Add more large, leafy salads and fresh fruit three days prior to your cleanse.

- Stock up on organic fruits and vegetables the day before you start.

- Increase your water intake to give your body a jump-start on flushing out toxins.

- Be positive about your upcoming cleanse—think of it as a gift to yourself!

- Determine how long you're going to cleanse. Typically, three to five days is sufficient.

Did You Know? *It takes only seventy-two to ninety-six hours for nicotine to leave your bloodstream, but nicotine withdrawal symptoms such as irritability, lethargy, dry mouth, insomnia, hunger, and dizziness can last up to a month, though two weeks is more typical.*

Now you know what measures you can take to make your cleanse as simple and painless as possible, but it's true there will still be some side effects, both good and bad, that you should expect once you start. Remember, these are perfectly normal, so stick with it! If you cheat even a little bit, you're defeating the purpose of the cleanse and wasting your time and hard work.

What to Expect During Your Cleanse

A cleanse is a great thing, but remember, especially if this is your first time, your body is going to be flushing out all kinds of toxins and "yuck," so some of the side effects won't be so pretty, especially in the first few days. The benefits of the smoothie cleanse far outweigh any side effect, so don't give up—you're doing yourself a huge favor!

The Bad Stuff

We'll start with the negative side effects first to get them out of the way and end the chapter on a happy note. The side effects from a smoothie cleanse aren't nearly as drastic as those you may experience on a juice detox, but still there are some.

Remember that you're forcing toxins out of your body, and the only pathways for them to leave are through your skin, your respiratory system, or your digestive tract. Therefore, you're going to experience some unpleasant side effects in all of those areas while your body is cleaning house.

- **Bad breath or body odor**—This is more prevalent with juicing, but you still may experience it.

- **Diarrhea or constipation**—You're changing your diet as well as cleansing, so a change in your digestive tract is probable.

- **Fatigue or energy fluctuations** for the first couple days.

- **Metallic taste or white coating on your tongue**—This is the sign of heavy metals and toxins leaving your system.

- **Mild headaches**—You're going to be getting more oxygen to your brain, so you may suffer a bit of a headache. You may also be experiencing withdrawal from sugars, caffeine, etc.

- **Mild rashes or acne breakouts** as toxins leave your system.

- **Nausea**—This shouldn't be too bad, especially if you weaned yourself off junk before starting the cleanse.

Though these are most certainly unpleasant, they aren't unbearable, and the benefits of your cleanse will soon become clear if you stick to your guns and see it through. The next section discusses some of the positive effects that you can expect from your cleanse.

The Great Stuff

Now that all of the negative effects you may encounter have been covered, it's time to discuss all of the good stuff resulting from your cleanse. After all, you wouldn't be doing this if it weren't an amazing way to clean up your body and get healthier, right? Consider this fact: at any given time, you're carrying around five to seven pounds of excess fecal matter just in your colon. Imagine how good it will feel to clean all that out! Here are a few amazing effects of your smoothie cleanse:

- **Beautiful skin**—Once all of the toxins are cleared from your system, your skin will look amazing. After all, acne is nothing but toxins leaving your body, so if you're clean, your skin is going to glow!

- **Improved cognitive function**—Now that your body is getting plenty of oxygen, and your digestive tract isn't sucking up all of the extra energy, you'll simply have a clearer head.

- **Increased energy**—Again, now that your body is clean and well nourished, you'll have a ton of energy.

- **Reduced cravings**—Since your body is being flooded with nutrients, and it's clean and functioning properly, you won't be craving foods to cure a nutrient imbalance. Also, since you stopped consuming all simple sugars before you began your cleanse, your cravings for those should be gone as well.

- **Weight loss**—This is the number-one reason why many people start a cleanse. Losing weight may not be the healthiest side effect, but it's certainly one of the most aesthetically pleasing.

Green smoothies provide all of the nutrients you need to survive, and by using them to cleanse your body, you're naturally infusing yourself with phytonutrients, enzymes, vitamins, minerals, fiber, and the healthful carbohydrates you need to function at your best. When your body is clean, it can more easily fight off ailments, such as cancer, cardiovascular disease, digestive disorders, and the signs of aging. You'll notice that you're slimmer, you look younger, and you feel better. So what are you waiting for?

In the pages to come, you'll find guidelines for three different cleanse schedules, as well as a collection of favorite recipes to get you started. Remember that if you cheat or give up, the only person that you're shorting is yourself. Think positive, picture yourself healthy, and then jump in with both feet—you won't regret it!

GREEN SMOOTHIE DETOX PLAN

To keep your green "meals" interesting and varied, include a combination of both sweet and savory. It's also a good idea to use a wide variety of produce to be sure you are consuming all of the nutrients your body needs. Otherwise, you may as well just reach for that cheeseburger! Smoothies are a great way to add nutrition to your diet or clean out your digestive tract so that your entire body can function optimally. The following section takes a look at a few different cleanses, discusses their uses, and creates a few sample meal plans.

One-Day Cleanse

Single-day cleanses are a fairly common practice and much simpler to complete than an extended cleanse. Though they don't offer the dramatic results of a longer fast, there are some definite benefits to sticking to smoothies even for a day. Some reasons you might choose a single-day cleanse include:

- You just want a nice burst of nutrients without grains or meats interfering with their absorption.

- You want to give your body a rest after a big eating event like a vacation.

- You'd like to see if cleansing is right for you and want to start slow.

Here's a sample meal plan to get you started:

Breakfast: Tropical Blast Booster

Midmorning Snack: The Mister Ed Special

Lunch: Peter Rabbit Cocktail Smoothie

Afternoon Pick-Me-Up: Cranberry Ginger Julep

Dinner: Blended Broccochini Soup

Feel free, of course, to mix these up or add to them if you're still hungry. These smoothies have a wide range of health benefits and flavor profiles, which will give you a general sense of what smoothie cleansing is all about.

Three-Day Cleanse

Many people enter the world of cleansing with short, three-day cleanses. This is a great way to sweep all of the accumulated garbage out of your digestive tract without really giving your brain time to go into deprivation mode. The three-day approach allows you to get your feet wet without turning the cleanse into a negative experience marked by cravings for solid food! Another great use for a three-day smoothie cleanse is to ease your body into a fast: some people start with smoothies for three days, then step it up to a more intense all-juice fast or detox. Regardless, if you'd like to try a three-day cleanse, here is a sample meal plan for you below.

Day 1

Breakfast: Tropical Blast Booster

Midmorning Snack: The Mister Ed Special

Lunch: Peter Rabbit Cocktail Smoothie

Afternoon Pick-Me-Up: Cranberry Ginger Julep

Dinner: Blended Broccochini Soup

Day 2

Breakfast: Plum Yummy

Midmorning Snack: Hidden Beauty Smoothie

Lunch: South of the Border Smoothie

Afternoon Pick-Me-Up: Lanky Limojito

Dinner: Slender Sicilian

Day 3

Breakfast: Fill-Me-Up Smoothie

Midmorning Snack: Doctor Away Puree

Lunch: Lean Greenie

Afternoon Pick-Me-Up: Hidden Beauty Smoothie

Dinner: Southwest Slim-down Gazpacho

Five-Day Cleanse

For those of you who really want to jump in with both feet, you could try a five-day cleanse. This is actually optimal if you want to thoroughly clean out your digestive system. Simply follow the menu plan for days one to three, plus the sample menu below for the final two days.

Day 4

Breakfast: Fruity Vitality Smoothie

Midmorning Snack: Super Berry Freshee

Lunch: Apple of Popeye's Eye

Afternoon Pick-Me-Up: Tropical Soother

Dinner: Summer Garden Smoothie

Day 5

Breakfast: Mega Omega Smoothie

Midmorning Snack: Plumarita Punch

Lunch: Immunity Endurance Smoothie

Afternoon Pick-Me-Up: Green Sweetie

Dinner: Salsa Soup Puree

Now that you have a few meal ideas, it's time to get started! You're going to feel healthier and have lots more energy because your body will be getting all of the nutrients it needs to fight disease and function at its best. So move on to the green smoothie recipes, an extensive collection addressing a wide variety of health issues.

(6)

GREEN SMOOTHIE RECIPES

Y ou've done your shopping at the local farmers market and now you have a refrigerator full of nutritious, colorful fruits and vegetables. The problem is, what do you do with them? Where do you start? Though there are no rules whatsoever when it comes to creating smoothies, getting started can be a bit daunting. Remember that your only limit is your imagination.

Regardless of whether you want to lose weight, improve your complexion, increase your energy, or just improve your health overall, smoothies can help you succeed in reaching that goal. To help you on your way, this chapter provides flavorful, nutritious smoothie recipes targeted to common conditions you may wish to address. Feel free to mix and match: just because a recipe is designated as great for weight loss doesn't mean that you can't drink it if you're already thin! All of these smoothies are delicious and packed with nutrients that are good for you no matter what your health goals are.

In the spirit of keeping things interesting, each category includes a couple fruitier smoothies and savory juices as well as one "soup." Enjoy!

Anti-aging Smoothies

The key to building your own anti-aging smoothie is to follow the "eat-the-rainbow" rule—include fruits and vegetables of all colors because they're packed with different antioxidants, phytonutrients, and vitamins that support healthful aging. Though this book's recipes focuses on green smoothies, note that a variety of other produce is included as well.

The Ailment

As people age, their bodies often don't function quite as well as they did when they were younger. Frequently this is just simple wear and tear, but as researchers learn more about the aging process, they're finding that many ailments previously attributed to getting old are more a matter of poor nutrition than anything else. For example, eating right can delay the onset of wrinkles, keep your skin looking young, preserve your brain function, and keep your bones strong. There are even preliminary tests showing that age-related cognitive decline and conditions such as Alzheimer's disease may actually be treated with certain foods.

The Cure

To keep your mind and body young and healthy, key nutrients to look for include:

- Vitamin A—This vitamin is known to help maintain eye health, lower LDL (bad) cholesterol levels, and fight free radicals that cause disease and physical signs of aging. Carrots, dark leafy greens, sweet potatoes, cayenne peppers, and red peppers all contain vitamin A.

- Vitamin D—Research is linking vitamin D to several different aspects of aging, including brain function and maintaining DNA structure by preventing telomere shortening. Since vitamin D is absorbed through your skin from the sun and cannot be found in fruits or vegetables, enjoy your smoothies outside. Getting ten to fifteen minutes of morning sun should do the trick; avoid prolonged midday exposure to prevent a sunburn.

- Omega-3 fatty acid—The effects of omega-3s on aging simply can't be summed up in a line or two; they're necessary for proper brain function, they promote heart, prostate, metabolic, and immune health, and they protect you from many types of cancer. These essential fatty acids can't be made by your body and must be obtained from dietary sources such as fish, raspberries, strawberries, broccoli, romaine lettuce, and greens.

- Resveratrol—A polyphenol produced by some plants to combat pathogens, it's a superstar in the anti-aging world because it's been linked to everything from cancer and heart disease prevention to reducing age-related cognitive decline. It's found in grapes, blueberries, bilberries, and cranberries.

These are only a few of the nutrients your body uses to fight the signs of aging, but now that you have a general idea, take a look at some recipes that can help you stay young.

Plum Yummy

Plums are an anti-aging superfood; they are proven to help with iron absorption, and the vitamin C gives a nice boost to your immune system. Finally, the antioxidants in this smoothie help fight cancer as well as wrinkles and other signs of aging.

- 1/2 cup water
- 1 plum, pitted
- 2 kiwis, peeled
- 2 cups baby spinach
- 6 mint leaves

Add the water, plum, and kiwis to your blender, and pulse for a few seconds. Add the spinach and mint, and puree. Garnish with a mint leaf and enjoy!

Yield: About 2 cups.

Youthful Italiana

This delicious smoothie is reminiscent of spaghetti sauce. The beta-carotene in the tomatoes, kale, and peppers are great for your eyes, and the antioxidants in all of the ingredients help prevent wrinkles. Garlic is known to fight off disease, and basil is rich in calcium. Kale is also an excellent source of brain-healthful omega-3s.

- 1 medium tomato
- 1 clove garlic
- 1 green pepper
- 3 basil leaves
- 2 kale leaves

If this smoothie is a bit too thick, just add water. It's terrific either for lunch or dinner. As a matter of fact, if you'd like to leave it a bit thick, it's great as a chilled soup.

Yield: About 2 cups.

Super Berry Freshee

The berries in this smoothie provide antioxidants that help maintain memory and brain function while fighting off wrinkles and disease. Bananas are a great source of potassium and vitamin B-6, both of which offer valuable anti-aging benefits. Finally, the resveratrol and other nutrients in the grapes add an age-fighting punch. This smoothie tastes fresh and delicious, too.

- 1 banana, peeled
- 5 medium strawberries, capped
- 1/4 cup blueberries
- 4 kiwis, peeled
- 1 small cucumber, quartered
- 1/4 cup water

Toss all ingredients in your blender and puree until smooth. Pour into a glass and garnish with a strawberry.

Yield: About 4 cups.

Apple of Popeye's Eye

This one's about as green as it gets. The antioxidants, vitamin A, calcium, and folate in this smoothie make it an anti-aging powerhouse, promoting good vision, brain health, and urinary tract health, just to name a few of its benefits. After drinking this smoothie, you'll feel like a spring chicken!

- 1 green apple, cored and quartered
- 6 asparagus tips
- 2 cups spinach
- 1 medium cucumber, quartered
- 1/2 cup water

Add the apple and asparagus to the blender, and pulse until they are in chunks. Toss in the remaining ingredients, and puree until it reaches the desired texture. This one may be a little chewy and will keep you full for hours.

Yield: About 3 1/2–4 cups.

The Mr. Ed Special

It's no wonder horses love this stuff: packed with vitamins, antioxidants, and minerals that help fight cancer, promote good eye sight and digestion, and help keep you mentally sharp, it's a glass of amazing!

- 1 medium carrot, with greens
- 1 green apple, cored and quartered
- 1/2 cup water
- 1 small cucumber, quartered
- 6 mint leaves

Blend the carrot, apple, and water on the "chop" setting, then toss in the cucumber and mint leaves. Puree to the consistency you prefer.

Yield: About 2 cups.

Digestive Health

Maintaining a properly functioning digestive tract is imperative to good health. If your stomach, intestines, or colon can't remove and process the nutrients from your food, there's not much point in eating it! There are several factors that contribute to a healthy digestive tract, including stress, exercise, drinking enough water, eating enough fiber, and taking in the right nutrients. If you lack sufficient water, fiber, or nutrients, your digestive health may suffer.

The Ailment

If you're suffering from gas, bloating, indigestion, constipation, diarrhea, or just a general feeling of discomfort in your belly area, chances are good that you have some digestive issues. Often, this isn't a rapid-onset type of problem. It may take years of improper diet, lack of exercise, and insufficient water consumption to cause a noticeable problem, but once you start detecting the symptoms, you need to take action before it becomes a serious health issue. Plus, why suffer if you don't have to?

The Cure

How would you like to go through an entire day with no bloating, gas, heartburn, or stomach cramps? If your only problem is that your digestive system is backlogged, then there's good news: a good cleanse will get you back on track in no time. Cleaning out your system is just the first step, though. You need to keep it clean, drink plenty of water, and make sure that you're taking in all the nutrients you need for healthy digestion.

Vitamins C and D are two primary nutrients you need—and don't forget that in order to properly use vitamin D, your body will need vitamins A and K, too. Also, don't forget the fiber! Keeping all this in mind, here are some great recipes to start you on your way to good digestive health.

Blended Broccochini Soup

This soup is packed with fiber that will clean out your digestive tract, and it includes all of the necessary vitamins to promote optimal health. Cilantro is an antibacterial, rich in gut-healthful minerals, which prevents nausea and relieves gas. This smoothie has a rich, spicy flavor that you can lighten up, if you need to, by adding an apple.

- 1/2 cup water
- 1 cup broccoli florets
- 2 kale leaves
- 1 medium cucumber, quartered
- 1 cup zucchini, cubed
- 3 small sprigs cilantro

Add the water to the blender first, then add the broccoli and the kale. Pulse until there are only small pieces, then add the rest of the ingredients, and blend until smooth. Serve in a bowl and garnish with a sprig of cilantro.

Yield: About 3 cups.

Peter Rabbit Cocktail Smoothie

Cucumbers are high in both water and fiber and have been used for years as a natural cure for constipation and stomach upset. The magnesium in the spinach relaxes your intestinal muscles and draws water into your digestive tract. Refreshing and green, the cilantro lends this smoothie a spicy bite.

- 1 carrot, chunked
- 2 leaves kale
- 1 small cucumber, quartered
- 1 cup spinach
- 3 small sprigs cilantro
- 1 green apple, cored and quartered
- 1/4 cup water

Blend all ingredients together in the blender. If it's too thick for your taste, add more water or more cucumber or apple.

Yield: About 2 cups.

Cranberry Ginger Julep

Cranberries have anti-adhesion properties that can help prevent ulcers, and ginger and mint have been used as natural digestive aids and anti-nausea treatments for centuries. This light, sweetly spicy drink is a pleasure to drink at any time throughout the day.

- 1 cup cranberries
- 1/4 inch slice ginger, diameter of a quarter
- 1 medium cucumber, quartered
- 6 mint leaves
- 1/4 cup water

Combine all ingredients in your blender, and pulse until the ingredients are small chunks. Turn up your blender and puree until it reaches the desired consistency.

Yield: About 2 cups.

Green Sweetie

Strawberries and bananas are great sources of soft fiber that gently clean your digestive tract while delivering a huge nutritional punch. Cabbage is packed with fiber but is best known for its ability to soothe ulcers. This fruity smoothie is delicious, and if you blend it well, you won't even know the cabbage is in there!

- 1 cup cabbage, chopped
- 1 banana, peeled
- 1 cup strawberries
- 2 kiwis
- 1/2 cup water

Add all ingredients to the blender, and puree until extra smooth.

Yield: About 4 cups.

Tropical Soother

Pineapple contains an enzyme called bromelain that helps your body break down and absorb protein, thus improving digestion. It's also full of fiber, as is the plum. The mint and cabbage are also known for helping with digestion. This smoothie tastes tropical and you won't even notice the cabbage.

- 1/4 pineapple, peeled
- 6 mint leaves
- 1 plum, pitted
- 1 cup cabbage, chopped

If your pineapple and plum are ripe enough, you may not need water, but if you do, just add 1/4 cup at a time as you blend the ingredients in the blender. Blend until smooth and enjoy!

Yield: About 3 cups.

Disease Prevention

The saying that claims you are what you eat is absolutely true. As you learn how your body works and what causes disease, it's readily apparent that you can keep your body healthy simply by eating foods that provide the vitamins, minerals, and nutrients you need to function.

The Ailment

There are a group of diseases known as "diseases of affluence," which research shows to be caused almost entirely by poor diets. These diseases include metabolic syndrome, type-2 diabetes, obesity, coronary disease, and many types (if not all types) of cancer. That's right—cancer can be caused by a poor diet. Eating large amounts of refined sugars and flours and other nutritionally poor foods causes sugar spikes, insulin resistance, and chronic inflammation that promotes disease. New research is even tentatively suggesting that Alzheimer's disease is caused by diet. Fortunately, diseases caused by eating a poor diet can also be avoided or even cured by eating healthful foods while eliminating the bad ones.

The Cure

Eating foods high in antioxidants helps your body fight free radicals that cause disease and signs of aging, such as wrinkles and dull skin. Fruits and vegetables are not only high in vitamins and nutrients, they're also low in bad fats and cholesterol and contain no refined sugars at all. In addition, they're great sources of soluble and insoluble fibers that keep your digestive tract clean, preventing such killers as colon cancer and liver disease. The bottom line? If you want to be healthy, eat your fruits and veggies. Smoothies are a great way to consume a wide variety of life-saving produce on the go, so drink up.

Salsa Soup Puree

The health benefits of this delicious, spicy, salsa-flavored puree are out of this world. It includes numerous cancer-preventing antioxidants, and the lycopene in tomatoes helps keep your vision healthy. The capsaicin in the pepper and the vitamin C in the lime and garlic help you avoid colds and maintain healthy digestion. To control the spiciness, simply remove the pepper seeds.

- 1 medium tomato, cored
- 1 medium cucumber, quartered
- 1 green pepper, de-stemmed
- 1 jalapeño, de-stemmed
- 2 cloves garlic
- 1/2 lime
- 3 medium sprigs cilantro
- 1 green onion
- Parsley, for garnish
- 1 teaspoon chopped scallions, for garnish

Combine all ingredients in your blender and blend until smooth. Serve in a soup bowl and garnish with a sprig of parsley and chopped scallions.

Yield: About 3 cups.

Plumarita Punch

This drink helps your body do everything from cure ulcers to prevent cancer. Plums also promote iron absorption. This delicious punch is fruity and zesty but not overwhelmingly sweet—you may not even notice the spinach and cabbage.

- 1 plum, seeded
- 1 green apple, cored and quartered
- 2 cups spinach
- 1 cup cabbage
- 1/2 lime

Simply puree everything together in your blender. If you'd like it a bit thinner, add 1/4 cup water.

Yield: About 2 1/2–3 cups.

South of the Border Smoothie

Avocados are rich in omega-3 fatty acids, which help you maintain brain health as well as fight cancer, depression, wrinkles, and a host of other diseases. Vitamins A and C are both powerful antioxidants, and this smoothie has a ton of each. Reminiscent of salsa because of the tomatoes and cilantro, this smoothie is both filling and delicious.

- 1 tomato
- 1 avocado, peeled and pitted
- 1 green onion
- 2 springs fresh cilantro
- 1/2 lime, peeled

Blend everything together, adding 1/4 cup water if you'd like it to be thinner.

Yield: About 2 cups.

Fruity Vitality Smoothie

Cantaloupe is incredible for your immune system, and kiwis protect the DNA in the nucleus of your cells. The raspberries are packed with disease-fighting antioxidants, and the iron, magnesium, and calcium in the spinach are great for you, too. This smoothie is a bit sweet and tart, and you may not even notice the spinach except as a background note.

- 1/4 cantaloupe, peeled and seeded
- 2 kiwis, peeled
- 1 cup raspberries
- 2 cups spinach

The cantaloupe and kiwis should provide plenty of juice to make the smoothie, but if you'd like it thinner, just add a bit of water. Blend all ingredients together and enjoy!

Yield: About 3 cups.

Immunity Endurance Smoothie

This is a well-balanced smoothie that has a touch of sweet, which complements the savory broccoli flavor. Among many other health benefits, this smoothie really gives your immune system a boost.

- 2 cups broccoli florets
- 1 medium cucumber, quartered
- 3 stalks celery
- 1 medium carrot
- 1 medium apple, cored and quartered
- 1/2 cup water

Combine all ingredients in the blender, starting with the broccoli. Pulse until it's in small pieces, then slowly add the other ingredients and puree.

Yield: About 3 cups.

Improved Cognitive Function

This section is all about what your brain needs to function properly. For this exercise, think of your brain as a car. If you want your car to get you where you're going, you need to maintain it, right? If you just keep running it as hard as it will go without any fuel or maintenance, it's not going to run well for very long. In order to keep your brain working well, you need good rest, plenty of exercise (both physical and mental), and a good fuel source. The first two are topics for another book, but this book addresses your brain's needs for fuel.

The Ailment

Going back to the car analogy, there are many different types of "breakdowns" your brain can undergo. It can simply run out of gas or need a new battery, or it can completely deconstruct. The good thing is that there are almost always signs before something bad finally happens, right? Well, it's the same way with your brain. Small signs that your brain isn't functioning correctly include:

- Anxiety

- Brain fog

- Confusion

- Depression

- Inability to focus

- Muted or exaggerated emotions

- Poor concentration

- Poor memory and recall

If you're experiencing any of these—or if you'd like to *avoid* experiencing any of them—read on.

The Cure

Many functions of the brain remain a mystery, but the more that is discovered about how it works, the more that is understood about the importance of hydration and a quality diet. Because the rest of the body works on the "garbage in, garbage out" theory, it makes sense that the brain does, too. However, people are learning that it's a bit more complicated than that.

Scientists are finding now that a poor diet may actually *cause* many of the disorders and declines that up to now have been written off as unavoidable or age-related, such as Alzheimer's disease, depression, and Parkinson's disease. On the flip side, eating a healthful diet rich in the vitamins and minerals your brain needs to function can keep your brain healthy and working optimally well into your old age. Since smoothies contain all of the good stuff and none of the bad, they are excellent fuel for your brain!

Look for such goodies as omega-3 fatty acids and antioxidant vitamins B, C, D, and E, because research is showing that people who eat foods rich in these vitamins score better on thinking and memory tests than those who eat poor diets. To take it a step further, an overwhelming percentage of people with Alzheimer's have low vitamin B-12 and D levels, which aren't found in typical Western fruits or vegetables. So get your D from sunshine and your B-12 either from supplementation or such foods as seafood, eggs, and dairy products.

Great Minds Gazpacho

The rich variety of omega-3s, antioxidants, brain-healthful vitamins, and phytonutrients in this soup will give your gourd a real boost. The zesty green flavors blend well together to remind you of a delicious salad or a tasty veggie sauce. You can control the spice level by removing the seeds from the jalapeño or omitting it altogether, though it lends a nice note to the soup. Drink it as a smoothie if you'd rather take it with you.

- 1/2 cup water
- 2 cloves garlic
- 1 medium cucumber, quartered
- 1 medium avocado, peeled and pitted
- 1 green pepper, de-stemmed
- 1 medium jalapeño, de-stemmed (optional)
- 1 medium zucchini, quartered
- 2 scallions
- Lime, for garnish

Add the water to your blender, along with the garlic and cucumber. Pulse a few times to cut them into smaller pieces, then add the next few ingredients. Repeat until all ingredients are added, then blend until smooth. Serve in a soup bowl, and garnish with a full lime twist.

Yield: About 4 cups.

Mega Omega Smoothie

Between the omega-3s that avocados offer and the proliferate amount of phenols, vitamins C and E, and trace minerals found in the entire smoothie, you can't get any more brain-healthful than this. It's mildly sweet and full of good fiber and healthful carbs, so drink this for breakfast or to get you through that midmorning or late-afternoon brain slump.

- 1 avocado, peeled and pitted
- 1 mango, peeled and pitted
- 1 pinch of cilantro
- 1/2 lime, peeled
- 1/2 cup strawberries, capped
- 1/4 cup water

Add all ingredients to your blender, and puree until it reaches the desired consistency. Since there are no flavors to hide, you may want to leave this one a bit chunky to get the satisfaction of chewing. Enjoy!

Yield: About 2 cups.

Focused Vitality Smoothie

The quercetin in apples has been shown to protect your brain from diseases such as Alzheimer's, and asparagus is packed with vitamins A, C, E, and K, plus chromium, a mineral that helps insulin transport glucose, your brain's fuel. The lettuce and grapes are nutritious and add a nice, mild flavor to this fresh-tasting smoothie.

- 4 stalks asparagus tips, tender halves only
- 1 green apple, cored and quartered
- 1/2 cup water
- 2 cup romaine lettuce, chopped
- 1 cup green grapes

Add the asparagus, apples, and water to the blender, and pulse until it's in small chunks. Add the rest of the ingredients and puree.

Yield: About 2 cups.

Mental Monkey Wrench

The vitamin C, flavonoids, and healthful carbs in this smoothie will really help keep your head clear and your thoughts running smoothly. If you like, throw in an avocado as well to get an additional boost of omega-3s. You're going to love the fruity taste for breakfast or as a pre-workout snack.

- 1 cup green grapes
- 2 kiwis, peeled
- 1 banana, peeled

Toss the grapes, kiwis, and banana into your blender and puree.

Yield: About 2 cups.

Beachside Breakfast for Your Brain

Vitamin C is great for memory, and this smoothie delivers it in spades. Since the spinach throws in brain-friendly folate, plus vitamins K and E, your noggin will love this tropical-tasting brew as much as you do!

- 1/4 cantaloupe, peeled and seeded
- 1 cup spinach
- 1/4 pineapple, peeled
- 1 orange, peeled

Toss all your ingredients into the blender and puree.

Yield: About 2 cups.

Increased Energy

Everyone's experienced it at one time or another—that dreaded energy crash. Energy drinks just seem to make it worse, and protein bars do help, but only for a little while. So what's the answer? Proper nutrition, of course. Just like with your car, if you don't give your body top-notch fuel—and plenty of it—you won't be able to function properly.

The Ailment

Perhaps you hit the wall around 3 p.m. and just can't seem to get through the last few hours of the afternoon until you can go home. Or does that brain fog and fatigue set in around 11 a.m., making it tough for you to focus on work? Regardless of when fatigue takes hold, it's never convenient. As previously discussed, your body gives you small signs before big things go wrong, and decreased energy is often one of them. In many cases, the cure is simple—you need to eat better!

The Cure

Simple sugars and pure carbohydrates are instantly turned to energy; they're the first forms of fuel that your body grabs because they're easy to convert. The problem is that because your body can burn them so easily, the energy you get from them is short-lived. One of the best ways to give your body something to burn long-term is to introduce fiber.

Because carbohydrates must be extracted from fiber before they can be used, foods high in fiber provide a great source of sustained energy. If you can get a bit of protein in there as a secondary source, then even better! Since smoothies are packed with fiber and plant proteins, they're great sources of steady energy, so grab your blender and keep reading!

Greener Goddess Gazpacho

The high content of healthful, slow-burning carbs, fiber, antioxidants, vitamins, and minerals such as iron in this soup will leave your body clean and your blood oxygenated, providing you with loads of sustained energy.

- 2 small bunches of watercress with greens
- 2 medium carrots
- 1 medium tomato
- 5 medium basil leaves
- 1 cup broccoli florets
- 1 green onion
- 1/2 cup water
- Scallions, for garnish

Blend all ingredients in your blender until pureed. If necessary, add more water. Pour into soup bowl and garnish with scallions. This recipe is nice to eat as a soup, or water it down a bit and carry with you as a smoothie.

Yield: About 3 cups.

Banana Berry Wake-up Call

Bananas are a great source of vitamin B6, fiber, and slow-burning carbohydrates that help keep your blood sugar steady. The arginine in watermelon helps keep you looking young, while the vitamin C in the pineapple, strawberry, and kiwi in this fruity, refreshing smoothie help keep you going, too!

- 1 cup strawberries, capped
- 1 banana, peeled
- 1 cup watermelon, cut from the rind
- 1/4 pineapple, peeled
- 2 kiwis, peeled
- 1/2 medium cucumber, quartered

Toss all ingredients into the blender and puree.

Yield: About 4 cups.

Green Island Goodness

There are only four ingredients in this tropical-tasting smoothie, but the nutrients it contains are out of this world! Arugula delivers energy-sustaining protein as well as the B-complex vitamins that your body uses both for short-term and long-term energy production. The potassium in the banana and high-fiber content of the entire smoothie keep your blood sugar stable, allowing you to sail through your day.

- 2 cups arugula
- 1/4 pineapple, peeled
- 1 banana, peeled
- 1/2 cup water

Add all ingredients to your blender and puree. The color of this one is a fun, bright green—enjoy!

Yield: About 2 cups.

Zesty Garden Greenie

Rich in biotin, thiamin, vitamin C, and even iron, this zesty salad-flavored smoothie will provide steady energy throughout your day, while fighting disease and brain fog. It's truly a glass of goodness with a taste reminiscent of a fresh, Italian tomato sauce.

- 1/2 cup water
- 2 carrots
- 1 medium tomato
- 2 cloves garlic
- 3 kale leaves
- 1/2 lemon, peeled

Add water and carrots to your blender, and pulse a few times to chunk the carrots. Add in the rest of the ingredients, and puree until it reaches the desired consistency. Enjoy!

Yield: About 3 1/2–4 cups.

Tropical Blast Booster

The combination of B-vitamins, minerals, iron, quality carbohydrates, and fiber in this smoothie make it a great afternoon pick-me-up. It's also delicious for breakfast, and you probably won't even taste the spinach over the delicious, tropical berry flavors.

- 1 pomegranate, peeled but seeds included
- 1 cup blueberries
- 2 cups baby spinach
- 1/4 pineapple, peeled

Add all ingredients to your blender and puree. If you'd like it a bit thinner, just add water, but its chewy deliciousness can make this smoothie extremely satisfying.

Yield: About 2 cups.

Healthy Skin

Everyone wants to have beautiful skin that's soft and free of blemishes or wrinkles. If you're one of the millions of people who think this isn't possible, then think again. It's entirely possible that many, if not all, of the skin issues that you experience are related to your diet. Acne and other skin conditions are the focus of intense research, and as more is learned about what causes less-than-perfect complexions, people are discovering that glowing faces may not simply be a blessing bestowed upon a beautiful few!

The Ailment

Acne, blotchy skin, wrinkles: many people deal with unhealthy-looking skin throughout their lives. Acne, originally thought to be caused by eating foods like chocolate, is actually caused by bacteria and environmental toxins. Your skin is one of three means that your body uses to rid itself of waste, and if you're ingesting a large amount of toxins without consuming foods that sweep them out, your body will push them out by default through your skin. Though there's no way to avoid toxins altogether, there are some steps you can take to protect yourself from these disease-causing poisons.

The Cure

It should be becoming fairly obvious to you by now that most of your body's ailments can be cured or avoided by drinking plenty of water and taking in nutrient-rich foods. Especially when it comes to skin issues, it's important to eliminate bad foods from your diet as well. To help brighten your complexion, look for foods rich in free radical-fighting antioxidants such as vitamin A, collagen-boosting vitamin C and magnesium, and healthful, moisturizing omega-3s. In addition, you'll need B-vitamins for producing new skin cells to replace those old, dead, wrinkly ones.

Green Vichyssoise

Potatoes are alkalizing and help balance the pH of your skin, which is one cause of acne. The sulfur and antioxidants in the onions and garlic are helpful, too. This soup tastes like a traditional potato soup, so feel free to enjoy it in a bowl for lunch or dinner.

- 2 red potatoes
- 1/4 red onion
- 2 cloves garlic
- 3 sprigs parsley
- 2 cups spinach
- 1 teaspoon rosemary
- 1 teaspoon thyme
- 1 cup water

Simply add all of the ingredients to your blender and puree. Serve in a bowl and garnish with a parsley and rosemary sprig.

Yield: About 4 cups.

Mediterranean Beauty Blend

Zucchini is one of those undervalued foods that is incredibly good for you. One of its benefits is that it contains proline, an amino acid that promotes collagen synthesis. This fresh-tasting, earthy smoothie is great as a soup as well, so enjoy it however you'd like!

- 1/2 cup water
- 1 medium zucchini
- 1 medium cucumber, quartered
- 1 green pepper
- 2 sprigs dill
- 2 springs parsley, plus more for garnish

Add water, zucchini, and cucumber to your blender and pulse. Add the pepper and herbs and puree. Serve in a bowl and garnish with parsley, or pour it in a glass for a hearty meal on the go.

Yield: About 3 cups.

Summer Garden Smoothie

Everyone knows that broccoli and tomatoes are good for you, but arugula has three grams of protein per serving, as well as potassium, magnesium, iron, zinc, folate, and vitamins A, B6, and C—all of the good nutrients your skin needs to be healthy. You can't go wrong with this smoothie—no matter what's ailing you—and the fresh veggie flavor will take you back to the delicious gardens of your childhood!

- 1/2 cup water
- 1 cup broccoli florets
- 1 medium tomato
- 2 sprigs parsley
- 1 medium cucumber, quartered
- 2 cups arugula

Combine the water and broccoli in the blender, and pulse until the broccoli is chunked. Add the rest of the ingredients and puree.

Yield: About 4 cups.

Hidden Beauty Smoothie

This is a simple, tropical-tasting drink, but don't let the lack of ingredients fool you. The three it includes are packed with potassium, vitamins C and A, and dietary fiber, which help keep your skin clear and soft.

- 2 cups spinach
- 1/4 pineapple, peeled
- 1 banana, peeled

Add all ingredients to your blender, and puree until the smoothie reaches the texture you desire.

Yield: About 2 cups.

Doctor Away Puree

Packed with vitamins, antioxidants, and amino acids, this smoothie will help keep your system clean while skin cells rejuvenate to give you a bright, clear complexion. Its lightly fruity, green flavor is pleasant to drink without tasting cloyingly sweet or overly green.

- 1 green apple, cored and quartered
- 2 kiwis, peeled

- 2 cups romaine lettuce, chopped
- 2 springs parsley
- 1/2 cup water

Add all ingredients to your blender and puree. Pour into a glass and enjoy!

Yield: About 3 cups.

Weight Loss

For many people, achieving and maintaining a healthful weight is difficult. Regardless of whether you have physical conditions that limit your ability to exercise, or you're stuck at a sedentary job where you work a million hours a week, it's never easy to make the right decisions on the run—which is why this collection of simple, nutritious recipes should make things just a bit easier for you!

The Ailment

Obesity has reached epidemic proportions in Western civilization, particularly in the United States. Much of this can be attributed to the widespread availability of quick, inexpensive, easy-to-carry processed foods that are high in bad fats and empty calories. Quite simply, it boils down to time and money. Healthful food takes longer to prepare and costs more money than unhealthful food.

The Cure

Fortunately, there's a solution that can help you slim down, fight disease, and live longer without spending an entire day cooking or a whole paycheck at the grocery store. Simple smoothies made with quality produce you can buy for next to nothing at your local farmers market are the perfect tools to help you build a healthful lifestyle on the go.

Southwest Slim-down Gazpacho

Hearty vegetables that are low in calories but high in fiber will help satisfy you and keep you full while helping you reach your weight-loss goals. The southwest flavors blend together to lend the gazpacho a tasty kick that's sure to be a hit.

• 2 medium tomatoes	• 2 cloves garlic
• 2 sprigs cilantro	• 1/4 lime, peeled
• 1 green onion	• Cilantro, for garnish
• 1 jalapeño, de-stemmed	• Lime, for garnish

Since this is a soup, feel free to leave it a bit chunky. You can control the spiciness by removing the seeds of the jalapeño, or if you prefer, replace it with a green sweet pepper. Simply blend all ingredients together, and serve in a bowl. Garnish with a sprig of cilantro and a lime twist.

Yield: About 1 1/2 cups.

Fill-Me-Up Smoothie

Grapefruit has long been associated with weight loss, and research backs it up. A combination of vitamin C and lots of fiber help you to burn fat while staying full. The potassium and other minerals in the banana, plum, and spinach assist with muscle recovery after a workout, and the fruity taste makes it delicious for breakfast or a snack.

• 1 grapefruit, peeled and seeded	• 1 banana, peeled
	• 2 cups spinach
• 1 plum, pitted	• 1/4 cup water

Add all ingredients to the blender and puree. Pour into a cup and enjoy.

Yield: About 3 cups.

Slender Sicilian

The rich flavors of this smoothie will remind you of a delicious spaghetti sauce, while the nutrients help your body fight fat, and the fiber keeps you full until your next meal. It's nutritious enough to drink more than once per day, because it offers nearly everything that your body needs all in one delicious glass.

- 1 medium tomato
- 2 medium radishes with greens
- 4 basil leaves
- 1 green pepper
- 2 stalks celery
- 1/2 cup water

Combine all ingredients in your blender and puree. With so many great flavors in this smoothie, you may want to leave it a bit chunky to enjoy some of them individually.

Yield: About 2–3 cups.

Lean Greenie

If you've been in the dieting world for more than ten minutes, you've most likely heard about the weight-loss benefits of cabbage and spinach. Toss in an apple to keep the doctor away and some kiwi just for extra vitamin C, and you've got a slightly sweet smoothie that will make you love green eating!

- 1/2 cup water
- 1 cup cabbage
- 2 cups spinach
- 1 green apple, cored and quartered
- 2 kiwis, peeled

Add all ingredients to your blender 2 at a time, starting with the water and cabbage, and pulsing between additions. Once all ingredients are in there, puree. Pour into a glass and enjoy.

Yield: About 3 cups.

Lanky Limojito

This is a great little recipe if you're looking for a light, refreshing cocktail. The citrus in it will help you burn fat, and the high water and fiber content will help keep you full and flush toxins and fat out of your system. Also, if you're looking for a low-calorie alternative to standard mojito mix, this is it.

- 1 lime, peeled
- 5 mint leaves
- 1 medium cucumber, quartered

Add all ingredients to your blender and puree. These flavors play well together, so if you'd like to leave it a bit chunky to enjoy chewing the individual components, feel free to do so.

Yield: About 2 cups.

CONCLUSION

Regardless of whether you're simply looking to add more fruits and vegetables to your daily regimen, or would like to address particular health conditions, smoothies are a great addition to your diet. If you hate the taste of vegetables but love pineapple, strawberries, and other fruits, smoothies are a terrific way to boost your vegetable intake without having to plug your nose as they go down. In a nutshell, no matter what your health goal is, smoothies can help you reach it.

You should now have several important points in hand to help make your smoothie-making adventure successful. Here's a review of a few guidelines, and perhaps a couple of new ones.

- If your smoothie tastes too strongly of vegetables, add in a cucumber, an apple, or some water.

- If your smoothie is too sweet, add a cucumber.

- Don't make more than you'll drink in a day, because fruits and vegetables begin to lose nutritional value soon after the skin is broken.

- Feel free to experiment with different flavors. If things get off track, see the first two tips.

- Remove the seeds and pits of apples, plums, and other fruits. Some of them contain toxins, while others simply taste bitter.

- You can control the spiciness of peppers by removing the seeds.

- Engage a buddy to start your journey with you—it's always easier to succeed when you have a support system!

Remember that adding smoothies to your diet isn't actually a diet; it's a healthful habit you're adding to your lifestyle as a long-term way of staying healthy, looking great, and improving your quality of life. With that in mind, find combinations of produce you truly enjoy so that you look forward to your smoothie. If it's a positive experience, it will turn into a habit that you anticipate and want to repeat!

Now that you're armed with some basic knowledge, tips, and recipes, good luck on your path to better health with delicious smoothies.

Made in the USA
Lexington, KY
08 July 2014